Table of Contents

Introduction

Living with chronic obstructive pulmonary disease (COPD) can present numerous challenges, impacting daily life and overall well-being. COPD is a progressive lung disease that includes conditions such as chronic bronchitis and emphysema. It is characterized by a persistent obstruction of airflow, leading to difficulty in breathing, reduced lung function, and a range of symptoms that can significantly affect one's quality of life.

The impact of COPD extends beyond the physical limitations it imposes. Individuals with COPD often experience breathlessness, fatigue, coughing, and frequent respiratory infections, making even simple activities challenging. This can result in decreased mobility, limitations in daily activities, and a decline in overall fitness and well-being.

While COPD is a chronic condition with no cure, there are various strategies available to manage its symptoms and slow its progression. One crucial aspect of COPD management is adopting a healthy lifestyle, which includes paying close attention to one's diet.

The role of diet in COPD management cannot be overstated. Proper nutrition plays a significant role in supporting lung health, strengthening the immune system, and managing the symptoms associated with COPD. A well-balanced diet can help individuals with COPD maintain a healthy weight, improve energy levels, reduce inflammation, and enhance overall respiratory function.

In this cookbook, we aim to provide you with a collection of nutritious and delicious recipes that are specifically designed to support COPD management. Each recipe focuses on incorporating lung-friendly ingredients that are rich in essential nutrients known to benefit respiratory health. By making conscious choices about the food we consume, we can empower ourselves to better manage our condition and improve our overall well-being.

It's important to note that while this cookbook provides helpful guidance, it should not replace personalized medical advice. Consulting with healthcare professionals, such as doctors or nutritionists, is essential to tailor the recommendations to individual needs and ensure the best outcomes for COPD management.

So, let's embark on this culinary journey together, exploring a range of flavors and nourishing recipes that will not only please your taste buds but also support your lung health. By adopting a COPD-friendly diet and making mindful choices, we can take control of our health and enhance our daily lives.

Chapter 1

Nutritional Considerations for COPD

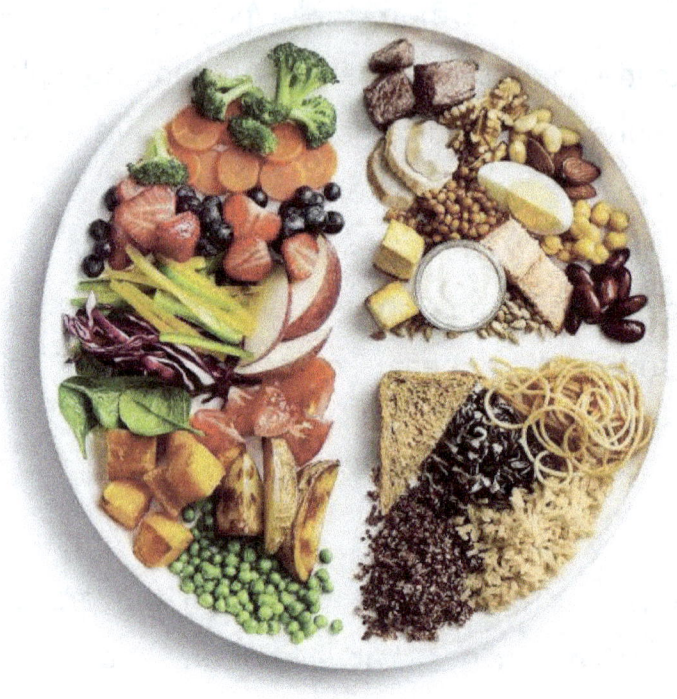

Maintaining a balanced diet is crucial for managing COPD effectively. The food we consume provides the necessary nutrients for our body to function optimally, and this holds true for individuals living with COPD. In this chapter, we will explore the importance of a balanced diet and highlight specific nutrients that support lung health.

Importance of A Balanced Diet

A balanced diet ensures that individuals with COPD receive the nutrients needed to maintain overall health and manage their condition. Here are key reasons why a balanced diet is essential for COPD management:

1. **Energy and Weight Management:** COPD can increase the body's energy needs due to the extra effort required for breathing. Consuming a balanced diet helps meet these energy requirements while preventing excessive weight loss or weight gain, both of which can impact lung function.

2. **Strengthening the Immune System:** A strong immune system is vital for individuals with COPD to combat respiratory infections. A balanced diet rich in vitamins, minerals, and antioxidants supports immune function, reducing the risk and severity of infections.

3. **Reducing Inflammation:** COPD is associated with chronic inflammation in the airways. Certain nutrients possess anti-inflammatory properties and can help manage inflammation in the lungs, thereby reducing symptoms and improving lung function.

4. **Supporting Respiratory Health:** Nutrients play a crucial role in maintaining healthy lung tissue and optimizing respiratory function. A balanced diet provides the building blocks necessary for lung repair, reducing the risk of

complications and enhancing breathing capacity.

Nutrients that Support Lung Health

HEALTHY DIET FOR COPD

- *Energy diet : Breathing effort increases energy requirements*
  - *Banana, avocado, pure cocoa, walnuts, non-refined oils*
- *Food with proteins in the main meals of the day*
- *Food rich in antioxidants*
- *Natural anti-inflammatories:*
  - *Aromatic herbs*
  - *Turmeric, ginger*

When planning meals for COPD management, it is beneficial to focus on specific nutrients known to support lung health. Here are some key nutrients to incorporate into your diet:

1. **Antioxidants:** Found in fruits, vegetables, nuts, and seeds, antioxidants

protect the body against harmful molecules called free radicals, which can contribute to lung damage. Examples of antioxidants include vitamins C and E, beta-carotene, and selenium.

2. **Omega-3 Fatty Acids:** These healthy fats are known for their anti-inflammatory properties. They can help reduce inflammation in the airways and improve lung function. Good sources of omega-3 fatty acids include fatty fish (such as salmon and mackerel), flaxseeds, chia seeds, and walnuts.

3. **Vitamin A:** This vitamin is essential for maintaining the integrity of lung tissue and supporting the immune system. It can be found in orange and yellow fruits and vegetables, such as carrots, sweet potatoes, and apricots, as well as in leafy greens like spinach and kale.

4. **Vitamin C:** Known for its immune-boosting properties, vitamin C plays a crucial role in reducing the severity and duration of respiratory infections. Citrus fruits, berries, kiwi, bell peppers, and broccoli are excellent sources of vitamin C.

5. **Vitamin E:** This vitamin acts as an antioxidant, protecting lung tissue from oxidative stress. Good sources of vitamin E include nuts, seeds, leafy greens, and vegetable oils.

By incorporating these nutrients into your diet, you can support lung health, manage inflammation, and boost your immune system. The recipes in this cookbook are thoughtfully crafted to include these lung-friendly nutrients, helping you achieve a balanced and nutritious diet for COPD management.

Remember, it's always important to consult with healthcare professionals or a registered dietitian to tailor your dietary choices to your specific needs and health conditions.

Chapter 2

Lung-Friendly Ingredients

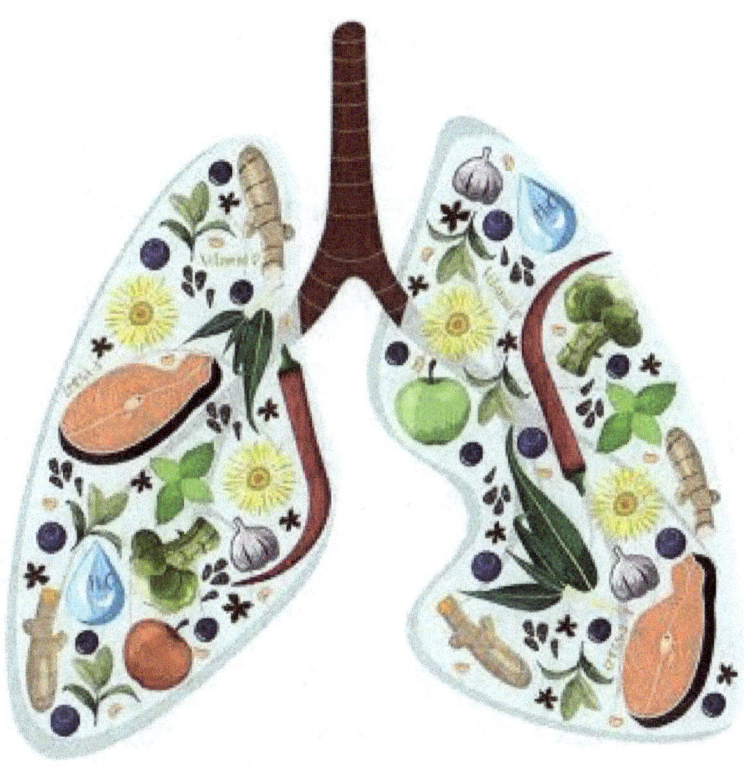

To support COPD management, it is crucial to incorporate lung-friendly ingredients into your diet. These ingredients are rich in essential nutrients that promote respiratory health and overall well-being. In this chapter, we will explore the essential ingredients for COPD management and highlight foods that are particularly abundant in antioxidants, omega-3 fatty acids, and vitamins A, C, and E.

Essential Ingredients for COPD Management

Including the following essential ingredients in your meals can provide numerous benefits for individuals living with COPD:

1. **Fatty Fish:** Fatty fish like salmon, mackerel, and sardines are excellent sources of omega-3 fatty acids. These healthy fats have anti-inflammatory properties and can help reduce airway inflammation and improve lung function.

2. **Colorful Fruits and Vegetables:** Incorporate a variety of colorful fruits and

vegetables into your meals. They are packed with antioxidants, vitamins, and minerals that support lung health. Examples include oranges, berries, kiwi, bell peppers, carrots, sweet potatoes, spinach, kale, and broccoli.

3. **Nuts and Seeds:** Nuts and seeds are rich in antioxidants, healthy fats, and vitamin E. Almonds, walnuts, flaxseeds, and chia seeds are particularly beneficial. They can help reduce inflammation, support lung tissue health, and provide essential nutrients for COPD management.

4. **Whole Grains:** Opt for whole grains such as quinoa, brown rice, oats, and whole wheat products. They provide fiber, vitamins, minerals, and antioxidants that contribute to overall health and respiratory well-being.

5. **Legumes:** Beans, lentils, and chickpeas are excellent sources of plant-based protein, fiber, and various nutrients. They can be a nutritious alternative to meat and contribute to a well-rounded COPD-friendly diet.

Foods Rich in Antioxidants, Omega-3 Fatty Acids, and Vitamins A, C, and E

To specifically target antioxidants, omega-3 fatty acids, and vitamins A, C, and E, consider including the following foods in your meals:

Antioxidants:

- Berries (blueberries, strawberries, raspberries)
- Citrus fruits (oranges, grapefruits, lemons)
- Dark leafy greens (spinach, kale, Swiss chard)

- Colorful vegetables (bell peppers, tomatoes, sweet potatoes)
- Nuts and seeds (almonds, walnuts, flaxseeds)

Omega-3 Fatty Acids:

- Fatty fish (salmon, mackerel, sardines)
- Flaxseeds
- Chia seeds
- Walnuts

Vitamin A:

- Carrots
- Sweet potatoes
- Apricots
- Spinach
- Kale

Vitamin C:

- Citrus fruits (oranges, lemons, grapefruits)
- Berries (strawberries, blueberries, raspberries)
- Kiwi
- Bell peppers
- Broccoli

Vitamin E:

- Almonds
- Sunflower seeds
- Spinach
- Kale
- Avocado

By incorporating these lung-friendly ingredients into your diet, you can provide your body with the necessary nutrients to support respiratory health, reduce inflammation, and enhance overall well-being. The recipes in this cookbook have been carefully crafted to include these ingredients, ensuring that your meals are both nutritious and delicious for COPD management.

Chapter 3

Breakfast Recipes

Breakfast is often considered the most important meal of the day, and it's no different for individuals managing COPD. Starting your day with a nutrient-packed breakfast sets the tone for improved energy levels, better concentration, and overall well-being. In this chapter, we will explore a variety of delicious breakfast recipes designed to provide essential nutrients for COPD management.

1. Overnight Chia Pudding

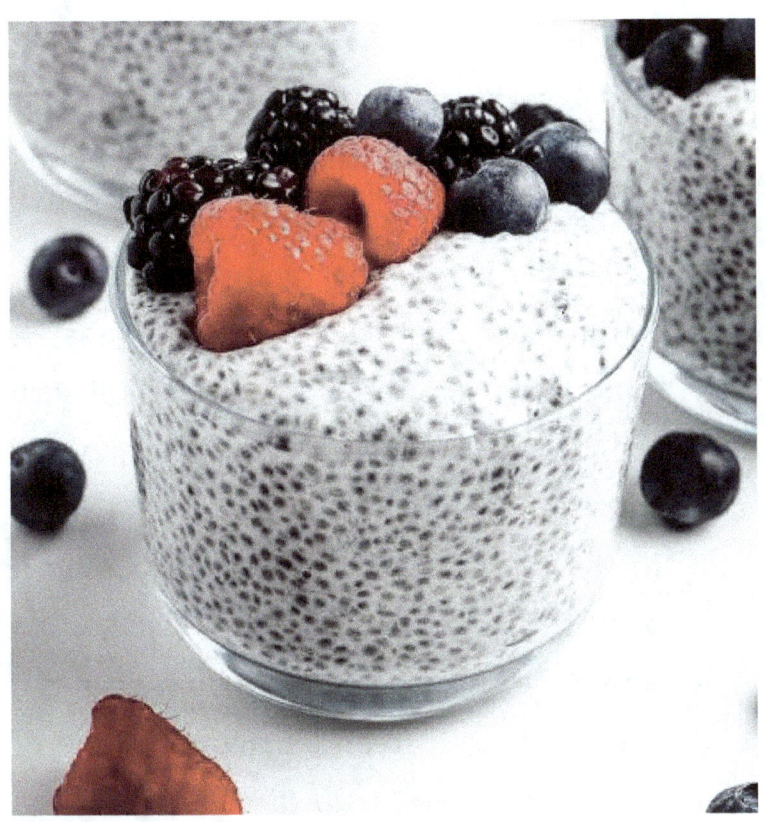

Ingredients:

- 2 tablespoons chia seeds
- 1 cup almond milk (or any milk of your choice)
- Fresh berries
- Honey or maple syrup (optional)
- Nuts or seeds for topping

Procedure:

1. In a bowl or jar, combine the chia seeds and almond milk. Stir well to ensure the chia seeds are evenly distributed.
2. Cover the bowl or jar and place it in the refrigerator overnight (or for at least 4 hours) to allow the chia seeds to absorb the liquid and create a pudding-like consistency.
3. In the morning, give the chia pudding a good stir to break up any clumps.
4. Serve the chia pudding in a bowl or glass, and top it with fresh berries, a drizzle of honey or maple syrup (if desired), and a sprinkle of nuts or seeds for added crunch.

2. Veggie Omelet

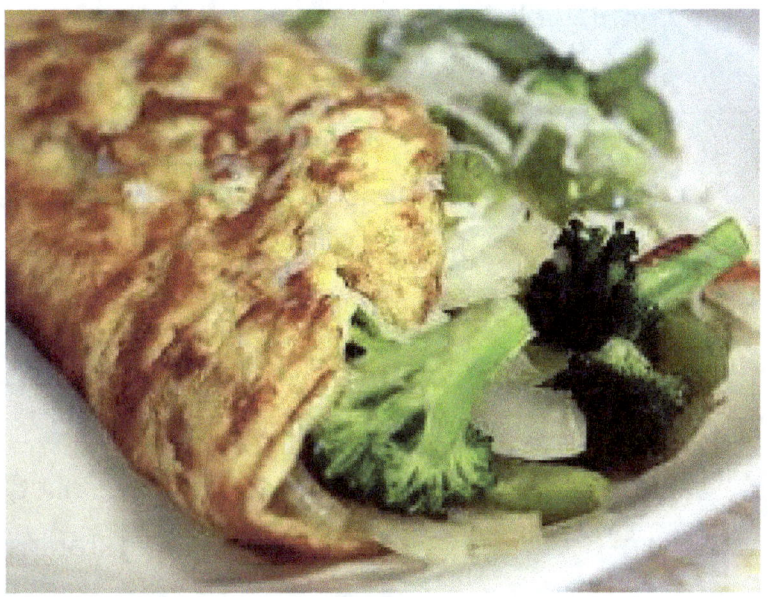

Ingredients:

- 2 eggs or egg whites
- Diced bell peppers
- Spinach
- Onion
- Mushrooms
- Grated low-fat cheese
- Salt and pepper

Procedure:

1. In a bowl, whisk the eggs or egg whites until well beaten. Season with salt and pepper.
2. Heat a non-stick skillet over medium heat and coat it with cooking spray or a small amount of olive oil.
3. Add the diced bell peppers, spinach, onion, and mushrooms to the skillet. Cook until the vegetables are tender.
4. Pour the beaten eggs into the skillet, ensuring they cover the vegetables evenly.
5. Sprinkle the grated low-fat cheese over the eggs and vegetables.
6. Cook the omelet until the eggs are set and the cheese has melted, folding it in half if desired.
7. Transfer the omelet to a plate and serve hot.

3. Greek Yogurt Parfait

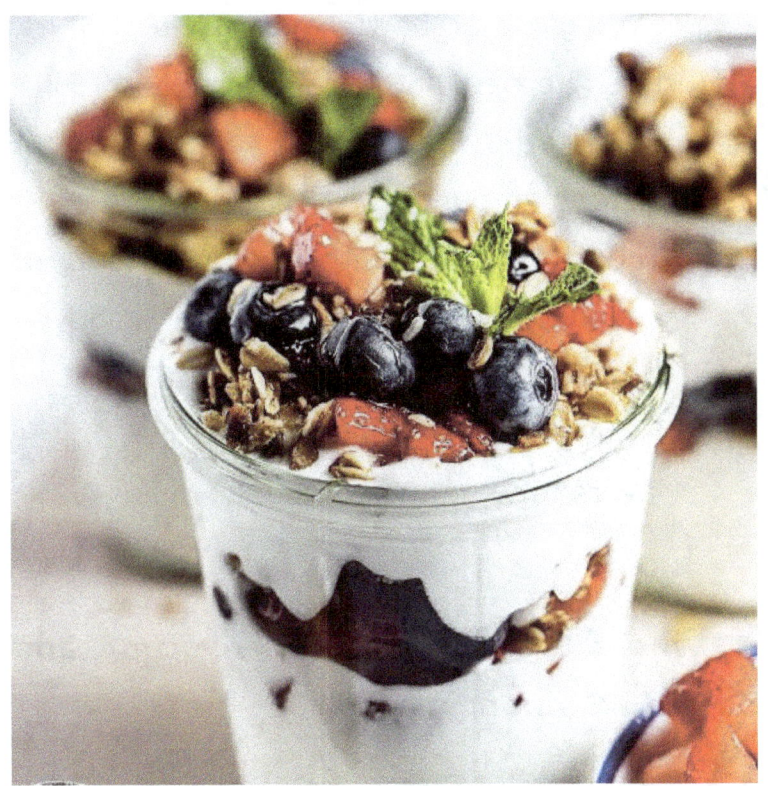

Ingredients:

- Greek yogurt
- Fresh berries
- Granola (preferably low-sugar)
- Chopped nuts
- Honey (optional)

Procedure:

1. In a glass or bowl, layer Greek yogurt, fresh berries, and granola.
2. Repeat the layers until you reach your desired amount.
3. Top the parfait with chopped nuts for added crunch and drizzle with honey if desired.
4. Enjoy the parfait with a spoon, mixing the layers together as you eat.

4. Whole Grain Toast with Avocado and Smoked Salmon

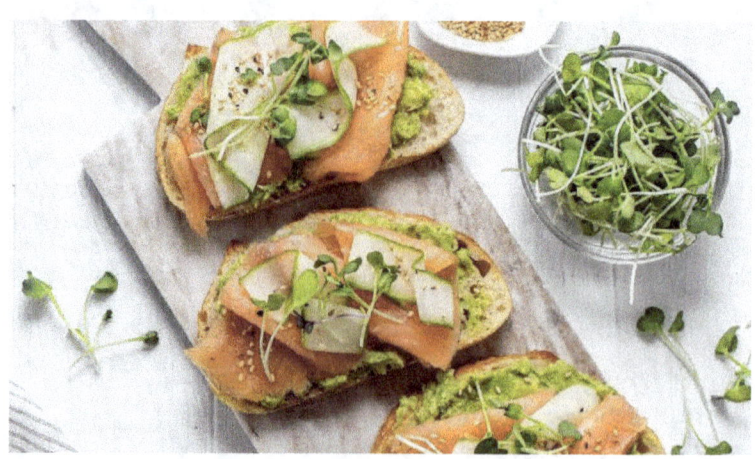

Ingredients:

- Whole grain bread
- Ripe avocado
- Smoked salmon slices
- Lemon juice
- Salt and pepper

Procedure:

1. Toast the whole grain bread slices until golden and crisp.
2. In a small bowl, mash the ripe avocado with a fork. Add a squeeze of lemon juice, salt, and pepper to taste.
3. Spread the mashed avocado evenly onto the toasted bread slices.
4. Top each slice with smoked salmon slices.
5. Garnish with a sprinkle of black pepper or a squeeze of lemon juice if desired.
6. Serve the avocado and smoked salmon toast as an open-faced sandwich.

5. Green Smoothie

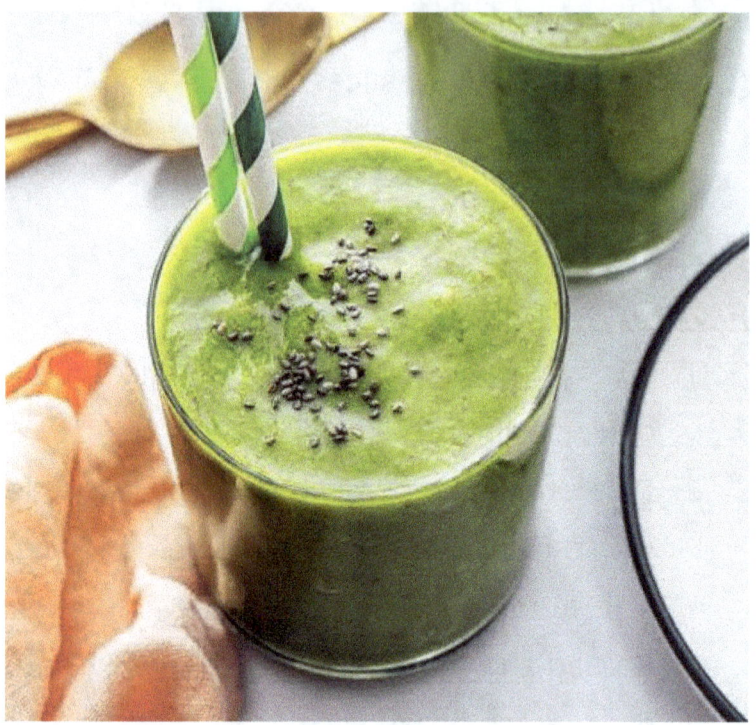

Ingredients:

- Fresh spinach or kale
- Banana
- Frozen berries
- Almond milk (or any milk of your choice)
- Chia seeds
- Honey or maple syrup (optional)

Procedure:

1. In a blender, combine a handful of fresh spinach or kale, one ripe banana, a handful of frozen berries, a cup of almond milk, and a tablespoon of chia seeds.
2. Blend until smooth and creamy, adjusting the consistency by adding more milk if needed.
3. Taste the smoothie and add honey or maple syrup if desired for added sweetness.
4. Pour the green smoothie into a glass and serve chilled.

These breakfast recipes offer a range of flavors and nutrients to kick-start your day on a healthy note. Remember to adjust portion sizes according to your individual needs and preferences. Feel free to experiment and modify these recipes based on your dietary requirements or personal taste.

Chapter 4

Lunch Recipes

Lunchtime presents an opportunity to refuel your body with a delicious and healthy meal that supports your COPD management journey. In this chapter, we will explore a selection of lunch recipes that are not only flavorful but also packed with essential nutrients to keep you energized throughout the day.

1. Quinoa Salad with Grilled Chicken

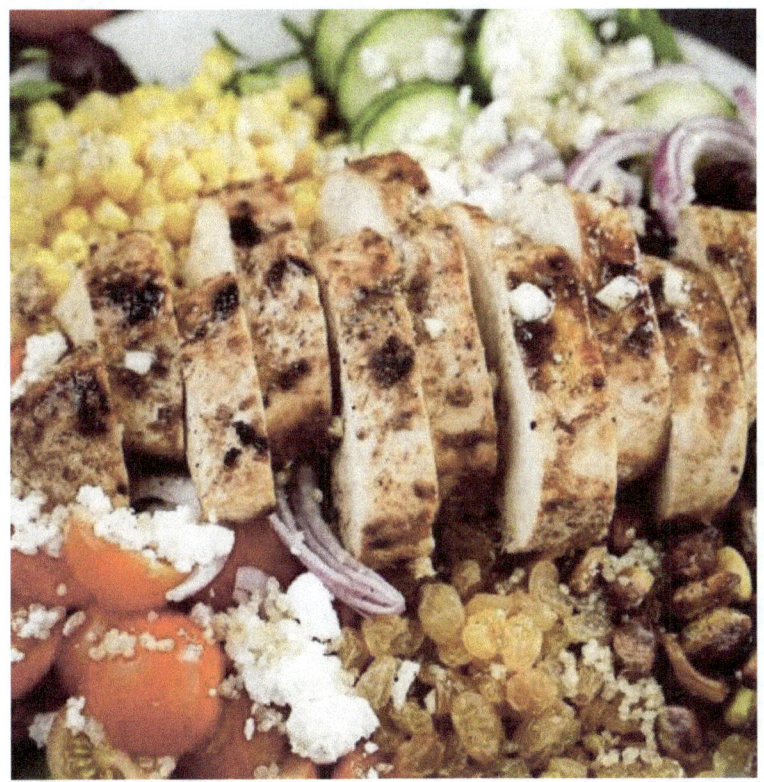

Ingredients:

- Cooked quinoa
- Grilled chicken breast, sliced
- Mixed salad greens
- Cherry tomatoes, halved
- Cucumber, sliced
- Red onion, thinly sliced

- Feta cheese, crumbled
- Lemon vinaigrette dressing

Procedure:

1. In a bowl, combine the cooked quinoa, grilled chicken breast slices, mixed salad greens, cherry tomatoes, cucumber, red onion, and crumbled feta cheese.
2. Drizzle the lemon vinaigrette dressing over the salad and toss gently to coat.
3. Serve the quinoa salad as a refreshing and protein-rich lunch option.

2. Whole Grain Wrap with Hummus and Veggies

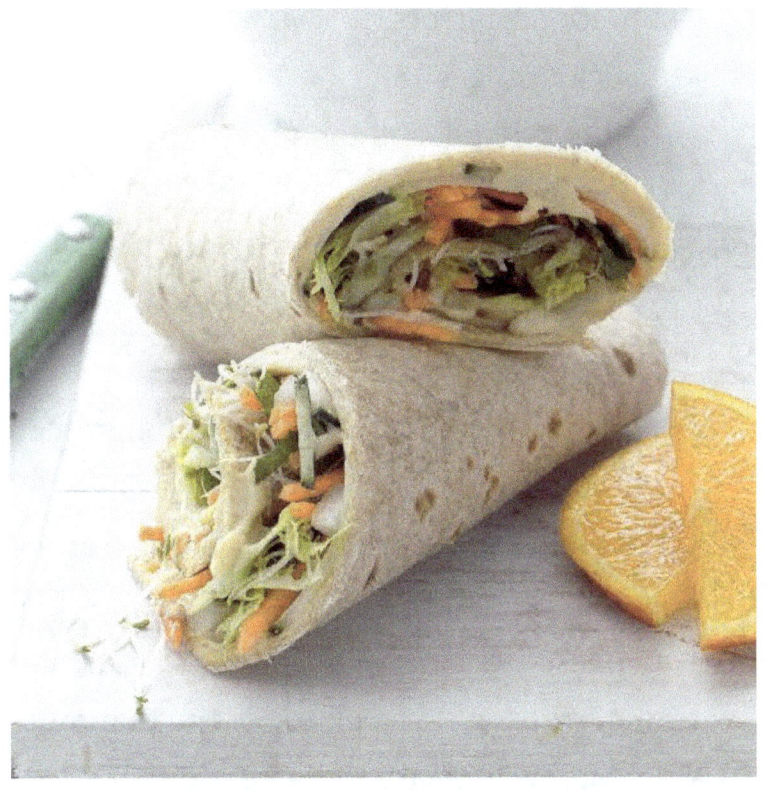

Ingredients:

- Whole grain wrap or tortilla
- Hummus
- Sliced grilled chicken or turkey breast (optional)
- Mixed salad greens

- Sliced bell peppers
- Sliced cucumbers
- Shredded carrots
- Avocado slices
- Salt and pepper to taste

Procedure:

1. Lay the whole grain wrap on a clean surface.
2. Spread a generous amount of hummus onto the wrap.
3. Layer the sliced grilled chicken or turkey breast (if using), mixed salad greens, bell peppers, cucumbers, shredded carrots, and avocado slices on top of the hummus.
4. Season with salt and pepper to taste.
5. Roll up the wrap tightly, securing it with toothpicks if needed.
6. Slice the wrap into smaller portions and serve as a satisfying and nutrient-packed lunch.

3. Lentil Soup with Mixed Vegetables:

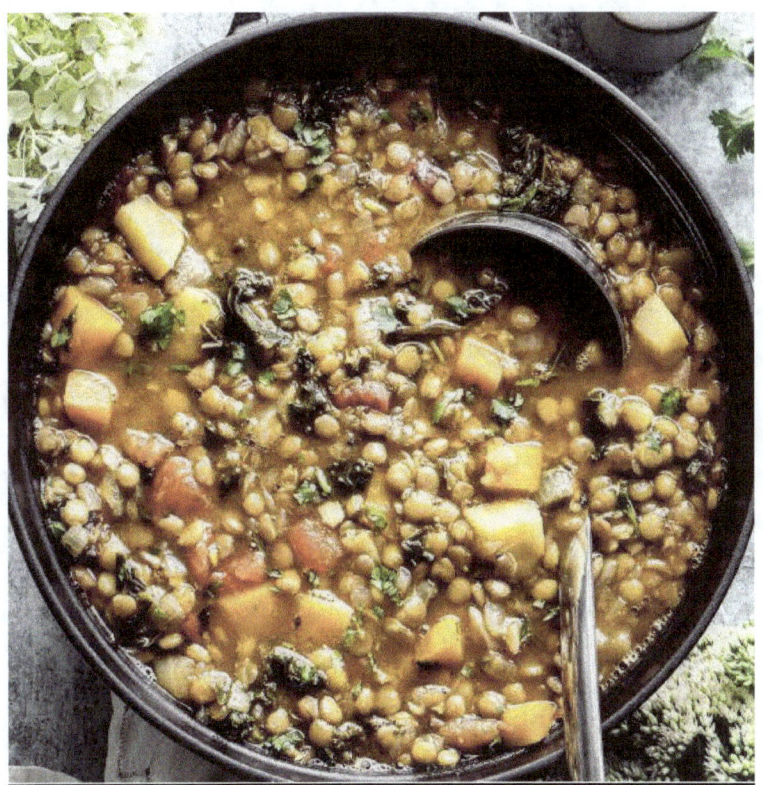

Ingredients:

- Cooked lentils
- Mixed vegetables (such as carrots, celery, onions, and zucchini), chopped
- Low-sodium vegetable or chicken broth
- Garlic, minced
- Dried herbs (such as thyme or oregano)

- Salt and pepper to taste

Procedure:

1. In a large pot, sauté the minced garlic until fragrant.
2. Add the chopped mixed vegetables to the pot and cook until slightly tender.
3. Pour in the low-sodium vegetable or chicken broth and bring to a simmer.
4. Stir in the cooked lentils and dried herbs.
5. Season with salt and pepper to taste.
6. Simmer the soup for about 15-20 minutes to allow the flavors to meld together.
7. Serve the lentil soup as a comforting and nutritious lunch option, ideal for colder days.

4. Grilled Vegetable and Quinoa Bowl

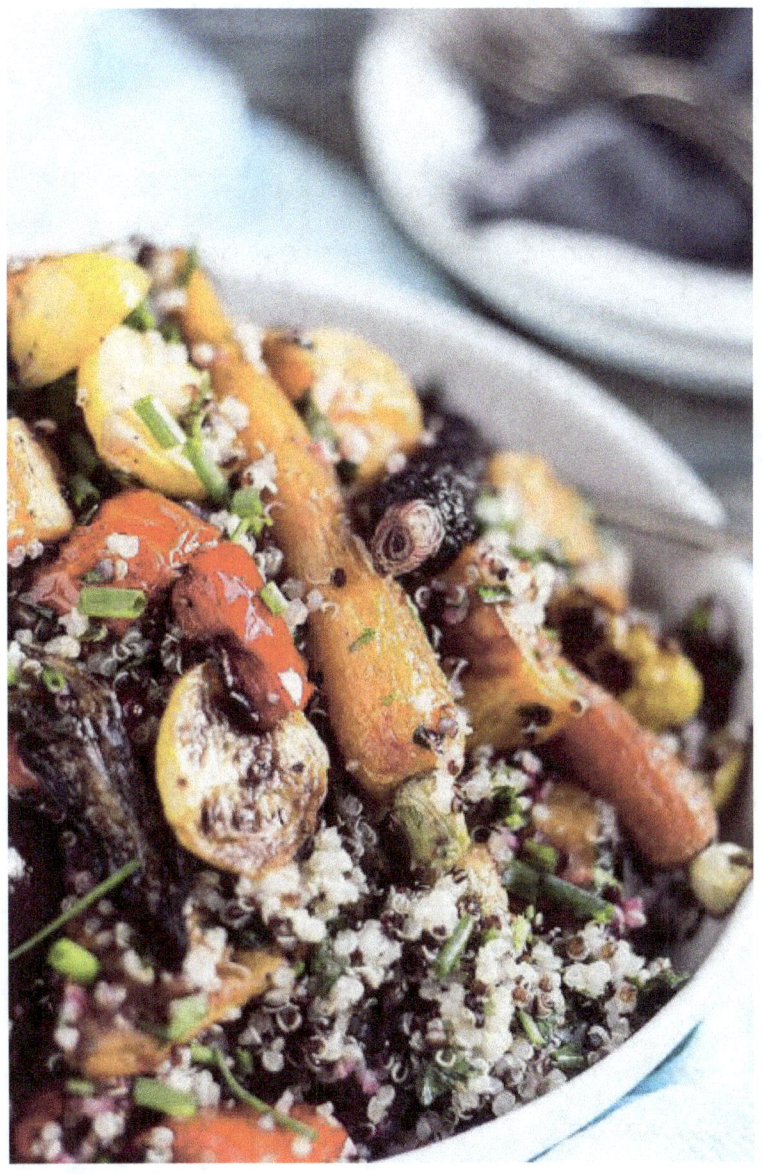

Ingredients:

- Grilled or roasted vegetables (such as bell peppers, zucchini, eggplant, and cherry tomatoes)
- Cooked quinoa
- Mixed salad greens
- Balsamic vinaigrette dressing
- Crumbled feta cheese (optional)
- Fresh basil leaves, torn

Procedure:

1. Arrange the grilled or roasted vegetables, cooked quinoa, and mixed salad greens in a bowl.
2. Drizzle the balsamic vinaigrette dressing over the bowl.
3. Sprinkle with crumbled feta cheese (if desired) and torn fresh basil leaves.
4. Toss the ingredients gently to combine.
5. Enjoy the grilled vegetable and quinoa bowl as a nourishing and satisfying lunch option.

These lunch recipes offer a variety of flavors, textures, and nutrient profiles to suit your preferences. Remember to adjust portion sizes according to your individual needs. Feel free to modify and customize these recipes by incorporating your favorite ingredients or adding a personal twist. A wholesome and tasty lunch supports your overall well-being and helps you stay on track with your COPD management goals.

Chapter 5

Dinner Recipes

Dinner is a time to wind down and replenish your body with nourishing foods that support your COPD management. In this chapter, we will explore a selection of dinner recipes that are not only delicious but also packed with essential nutrients to promote your overall well-being.

1. Baked Salmon with Roasted Vegetables

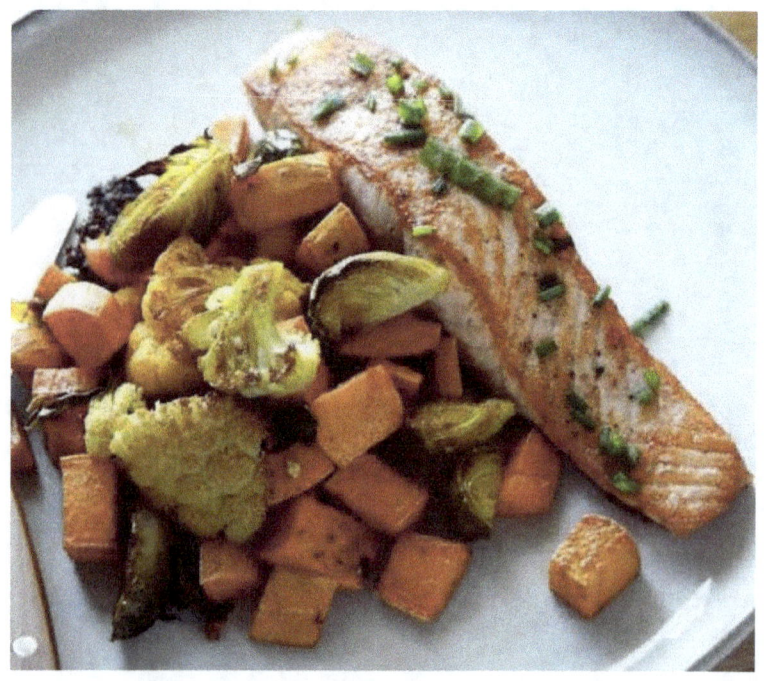

Ingredients:

- Fresh salmon fillets
- Assorted vegetables (such as broccoli, carrots, and Brussels sprouts), chopped
- Olive oil
- Lemon juice
- Garlic powder
- Dried herbs (such as dill or thyme)
- Salt and pepper to taste

Procedure:

1. Preheat the oven to 400°F (200°C).
2. Place the salmon fillets on a baking sheet lined with parchment paper.
3. Drizzle the salmon with olive oil and lemon juice.
4. Sprinkle with garlic powder, dried herbs, salt, and pepper.
5. In a separate baking dish, toss the chopped vegetables with olive oil, salt, and pepper.
6. Place both the salmon and vegetables in the preheated oven and bake for about

15-20 minutes, or until the salmon is cooked through and the vegetables are tender.

7. Serve the baked salmon with roasted vegetables for a flavorful and nutrient-rich dinner.

2. Quinoa Stuffed Bell Peppers

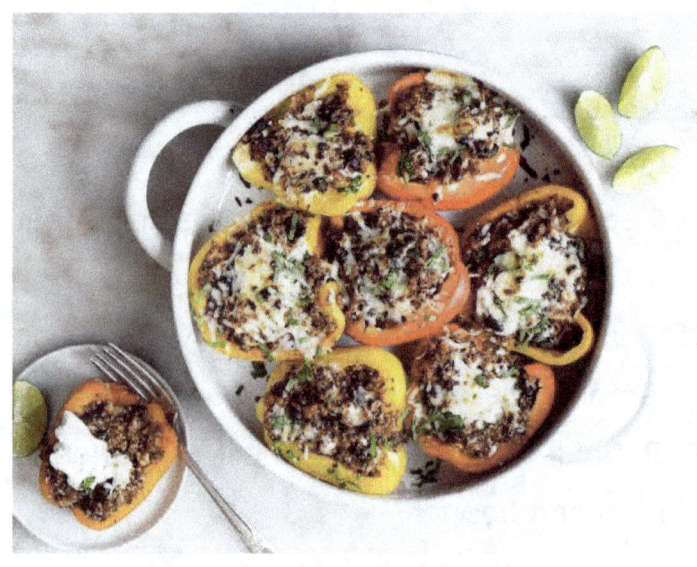

Ingredients:

- Bell peppers

- Cooked quinoa
- Ground turkey or lean ground beef
- Onion, diced
- Garlic, minced
- Tomato sauce
- Low-sodium vegetable or chicken broth
- Italian seasoning
- Salt and pepper to taste

Procedure:

1. Preheat the oven to 375°F (190°C).
2. Cut the tops off the bell peppers and remove the seeds and membranes.
3. In a skillet, cook the ground turkey or lean ground beef until browned. Add the diced onion and minced garlic and cook until softened.
4. Stir in the cooked quinoa, tomato sauce, low-sodium vegetable or chicken broth, Italian seasoning, salt, and pepper. Cook for a few minutes to allow the flavors to meld together.

5. Stuff the bell peppers with the quinoa and meat mixture, packing it tightly.
6. Place the stuffed bell peppers in a baking dish and cover with foil.
7. Bake for approximately 30-40 minutes, or until the peppers are tender and the filling is heated through.
8. Serve the quinoa stuffed bell peppers as a satisfying and nutrient-packed dinner.

3. Grilled Chicken and Vegetable Skewers

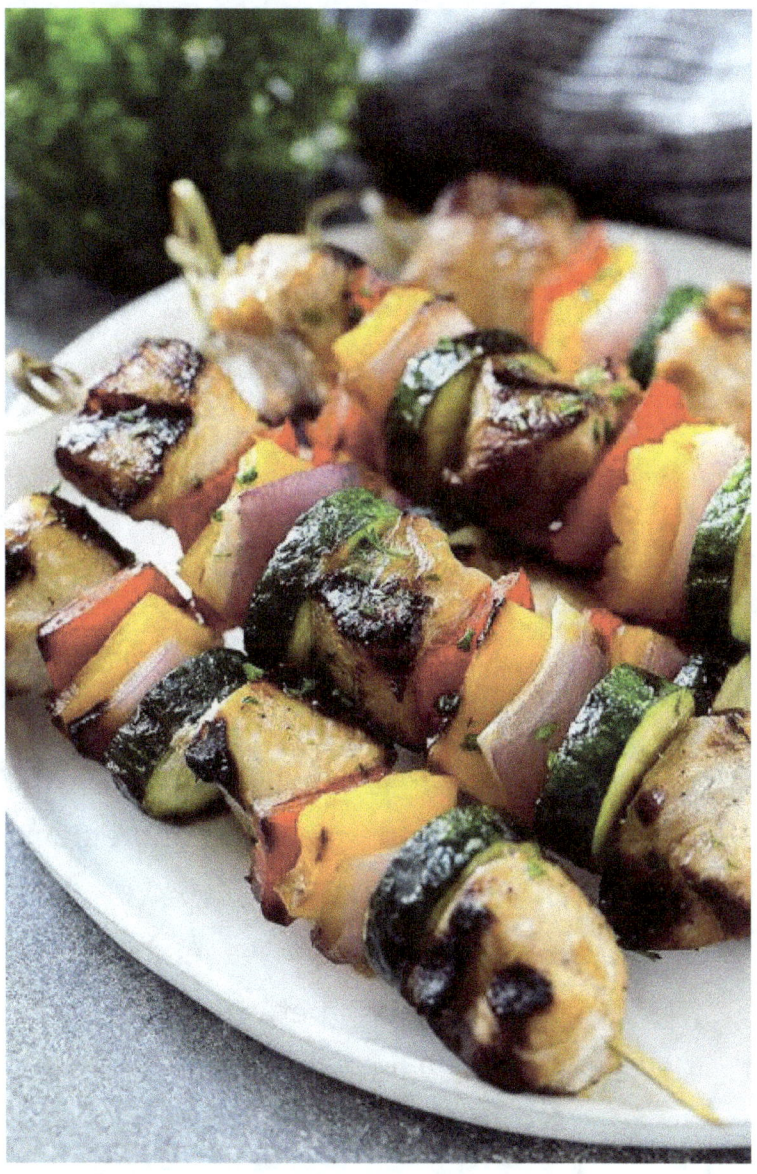

Ingredients:

- Chicken breast, cut into chunks
- Assorted vegetables (such as bell peppers, zucchini, and cherry tomatoes), cut into pieces
- Olive oil
- Lemon juice
- Garlic, minced
- Dried herbs (such as rosemary or thyme)
- Salt and pepper to taste

Procedure:

1. Preheat the grill to medium heat.
2. In a bowl, combine the chicken breast chunks, vegetables, olive oil, lemon juice, minced garlic, dried herbs, salt, and pepper. Toss to coat the ingredients evenly.
3. Thread the chicken and vegetables onto skewers, alternating between them.
4. Place the skewers on the preheated grill and cook for about 10-15 minutes, turning occasionally, until the chicken is

cooked through and the vegetables are slightly charred.

5. Remove the skewers from the grill and let them rest for a few minutes before serving.

6. Enjoy the grilled chicken and vegetable skewers as a protein-packed and flavorful dinner option.

4. Lentil and Vegetable Stir-Fry

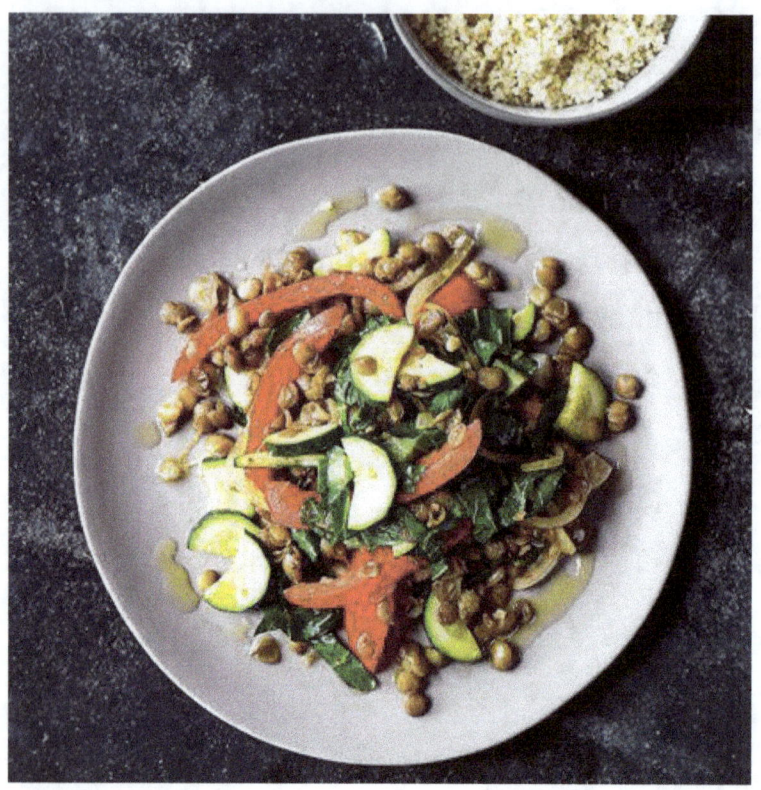

Ingredients:

- Cooked lentils
- Assorted vegetables (such as broccoli, bell peppers, snap peas, and carrots), sliced
- Garlic, minced
- Low-sodium soy sauce
- Sesame oil

- Ginger, grated
- Red pepper flakes (optional)
- Salt and pepper to taste

Procedure:

1. In a large skillet or wok, heat the sesame oil over medium-high heat.
2. Add the minced garlic, grated ginger, and red pepper flakes (if using). Cook for about a minute until fragrant.
3. Add the sliced vegetables to the skillet and stir-fry for a few minutes until they are crisp-tender.
4. Stir in the cooked lentils and season with low-sodium soy sauce, salt, and pepper.
5. Continue to stir-fry for another couple of minutes until the flavors are well combined and the vegetables are cooked to your liking.
6. Serve the lentil and vegetable stir-fry as a satisfying and fiber-rich dinner option.
7. These dinner recipes offer a variety of flavors, textures, and nutrient profiles to

suit your preferences. Remember to adjust portion sizes according to your individual needs. Feel free to customize these recipes by adding your favorite herbs, spices, or additional vegetables. A nourishing dinner supports your COPD management goals and helps you end the day on a satisfying note.

Chapter 6

Snack Recipes

Snacks are an important part of maintaining energy levels and satiety throughout the day, especially when managing COPD. In this chapter, we will explore a selection of lung-friendly snack recipes that are not only delicious but also provide a boost of nutrients to support your well-being.

1. Apple Slices with Almond Butter

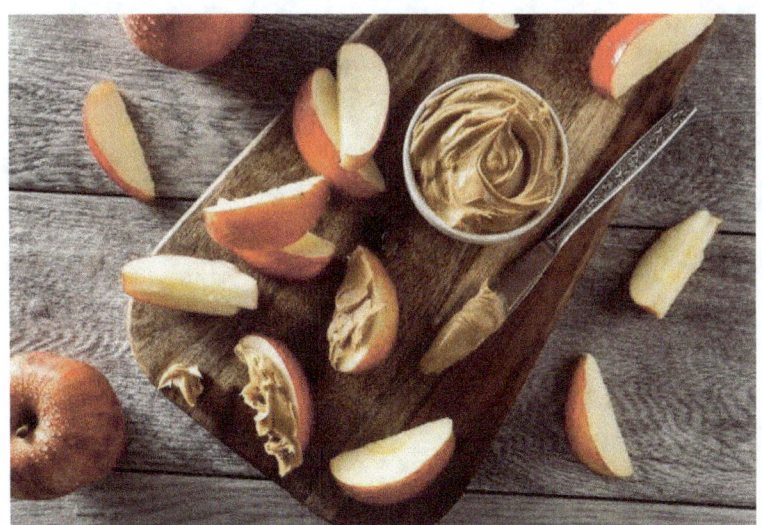

Ingredients:

- Fresh apple, sliced
- Almond butter

Procedure:

1. Slice the fresh apple into thin wedges.
2. Spread a generous amount of almond butter onto each apple slice.
3. Enjoy the apple slices with almond butter as a satisfying and nutrient-rich snack option.

2. Veggie Sticks with Hummus

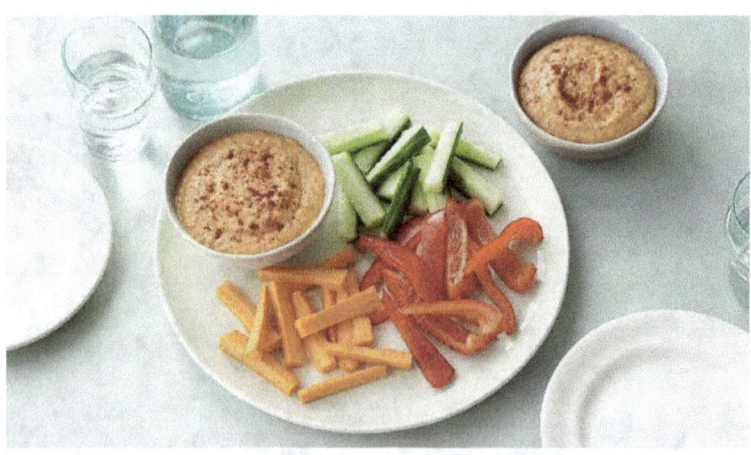

Ingredients:

- Assorted raw vegetables (such as carrot sticks, celery sticks, bell pepper strips, and cucumber slices)
- Hummus

Procedure:

1. Wash and cut the vegetables into stick or slice shapes.
2. Serve the veggie sticks with a side of hummus for a crunchy and nutritious snack.

3. Greek Yogurt with Berries

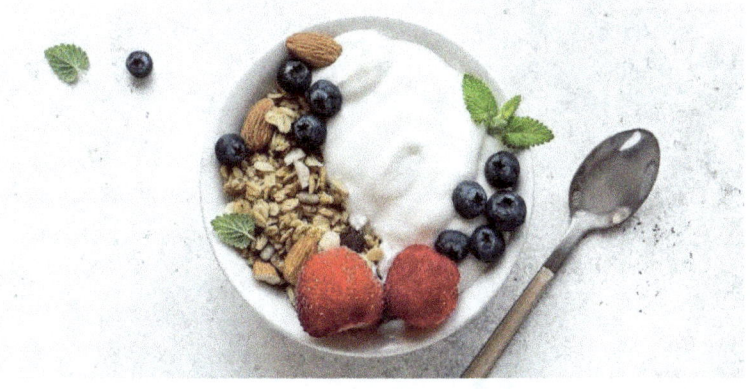

Ingredients:

- Greek yogurt
- Fresh berries (such as strawberries, blueberries, or raspberries)
- Honey (optional)

Procedure:

1. Spoon Greek yogurt into a bowl or small cup.
2. Top the yogurt with fresh berries.
3. Drizzle with honey for added sweetness if desired.
4. Enjoy the Greek yogurt with berries as a protein-packed and antioxidant-rich snack.

4. Trail Mix

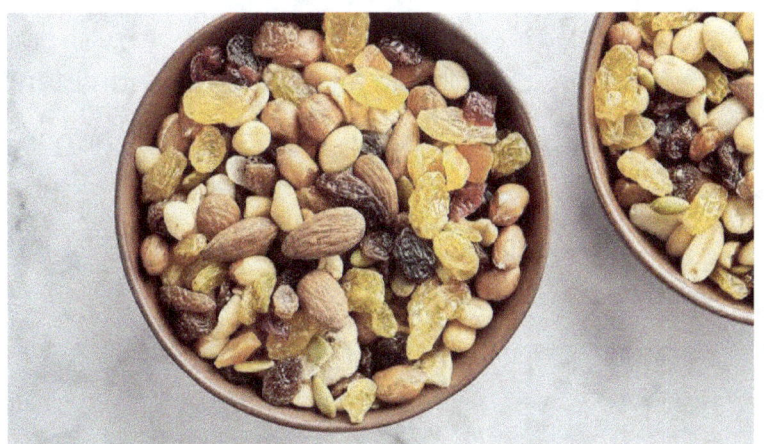

Ingredients:

- Raw nuts (such as almonds, walnuts, or cashews)
- Dried fruits (such as raisins, cranberries, or apricots)
- Pumpkin seeds
- Dark chocolate chips (optional)

Procedure:

1. Combine equal parts of raw nuts, dried fruits, pumpkin seeds, and dark chocolate chips (if using) in a bowl.

2. Mix well to create a balanced and flavorful trail mix.

3. Portion out the trail mix into individual snack bags for easy grab-and-go options.

5. Avocado Toast

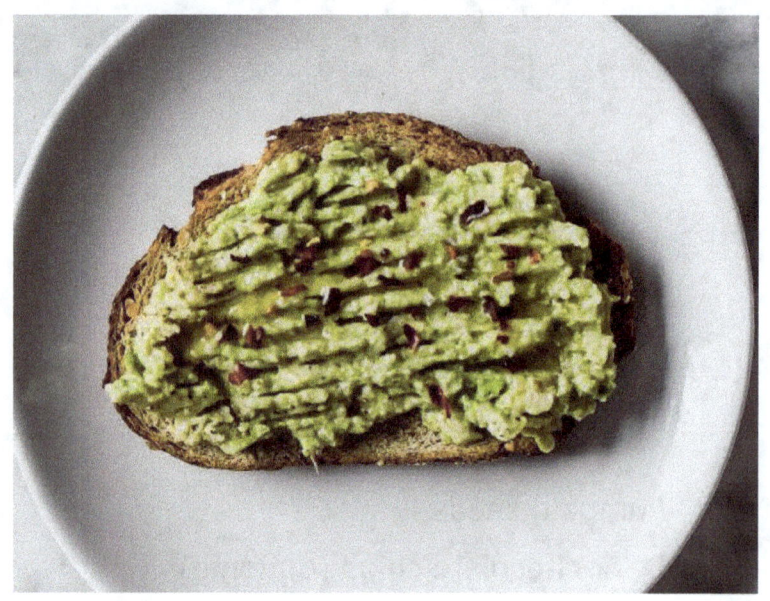

Ingredients:

- Whole grain bread
- Ripe avocado
- Lemon juice
- Salt and pepper

Procedure:

1. Toast the whole grain bread slices until golden and crisp.
2. In a small bowl, mash the ripe avocado with a fork. Add a squeeze of lemon juice, salt, and pepper to taste.
3. Spread the mashed avocado evenly onto the toasted bread slices.
4. Sprinkle with additional salt and pepper if desired.
5. Enjoy the avocado toast as a nutrient-packed and satisfying snack.

These snack recipes offer a range of flavors and nutrient profiles to keep you energized and satisfied between meals. Remember to adjust portion sizes according to your individual needs and preferences. Feel free to experiment with different combinations of fruits, vegetables, and spreads to customize your lung-friendly snacks.

Chapter 7

Beverage Recipes

Staying hydrated is essential for overall well-being and managing COPD. In this chapter, we will explore a selection of refreshing and nutritious beverage recipes that can help quench your thirst while providing additional health benefits.

1. Green Smoothie

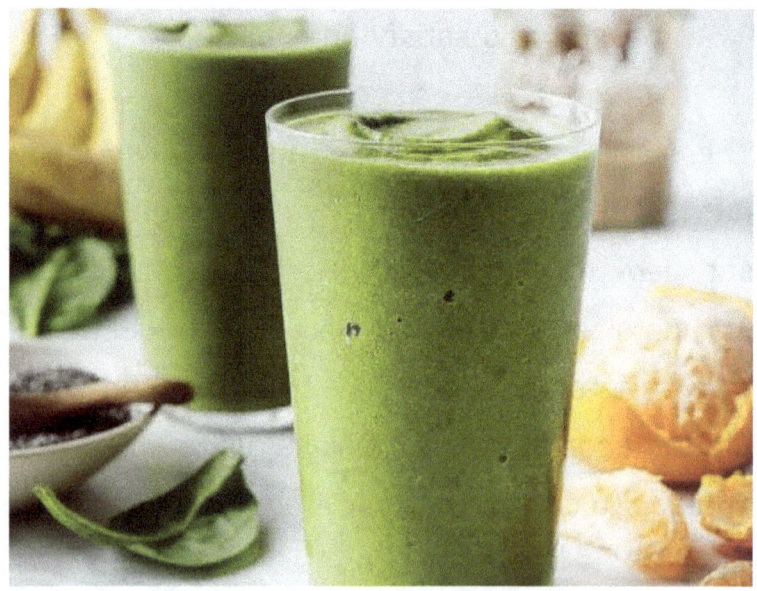

Ingredients:

- Fresh spinach or kale
- Ripe banana
- Frozen berries (such as blueberries or strawberries)
- Almond milk or coconut water
- Chia seeds (optional)

Procedure:

1. In a blender, combine a handful of fresh spinach or kale, one ripe banana, a handful of frozen berries, a cup of almond milk or coconut water, and a tablespoon of chia seeds (optional).
2. Blend until smooth and creamy, adjusting the consistency by adding more liquid if needed.
3. Pour the green smoothie into a glass and serve chilled.

2. Citrus Infused Water

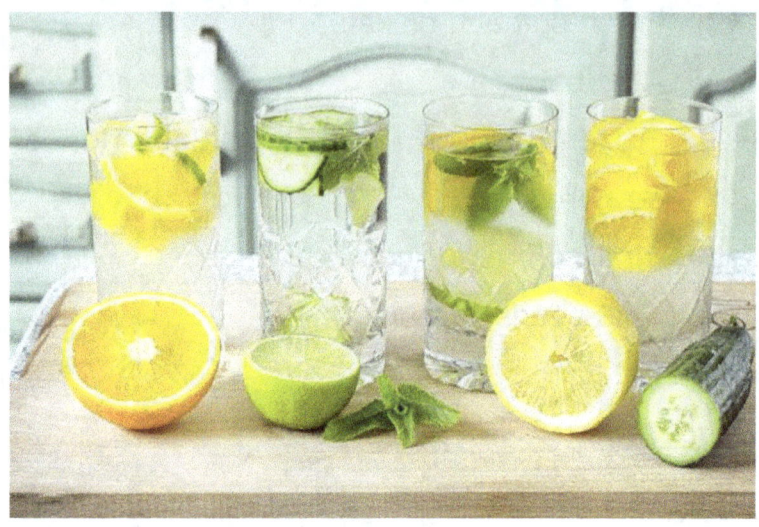

Ingredients:

- Fresh citrus fruits (such as lemon, lime, or orange)
- Fresh mint leaves (optional)
- Water

Procedure:

1. Slice the citrus fruits into thin rounds or wedges.
2. Fill a pitcher or water bottle with water.
3. Add the citrus slices and fresh mint leaves (if using) to the water.

4. Allow the water to infuse for at least 30 minutes to enhance the flavors.
5. Serve the citrus infused water over ice for a refreshing and hydrating beverage.

3. Herbal Iced Tea

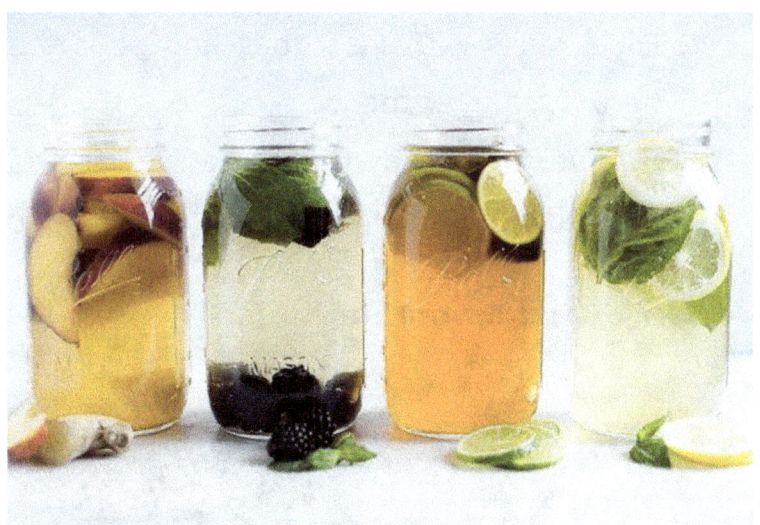

<u>Ingredients:</u>

- Herbal tea bags (such as chamomile, peppermint, or ginger)
- Fresh lemon slices
- Honey or stevia (optional)
- Ice cubes

Procedure:

1. Brew herbal tea bags according to the package instructions.
2. Allow the tea to cool to room temperature.
3. Add fresh lemon slices and sweeten with honey or stevia if desired.
4. Fill a glass with ice cubes and pour the herbal tea over the ice.
5. Stir well and enjoy the herbal iced tea as a soothing and flavorful beverage.

4. Berry Blast Smoothie

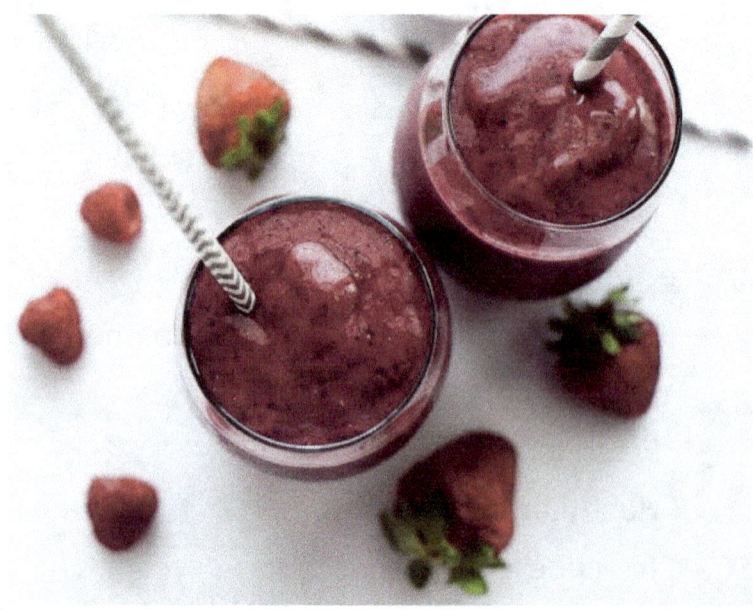

Ingredients:

- Frozen mixed berries (such as raspberries, blueberries, and strawberries)
- Greek yogurt or almond milk
- Honey or maple syrup (optional)
- Ice cubes

Procedure:

1. In a blender, combine a handful of frozen mixed berries, a dollop of Greek yogurt or a splash of almond milk, and sweeten with honey or maple syrup if desired.
2. Add ice cubes to achieve the desired thickness and blend until smooth.
3. Pour the berry blast smoothie into a glass and serve chilled.

5. Golden Milk

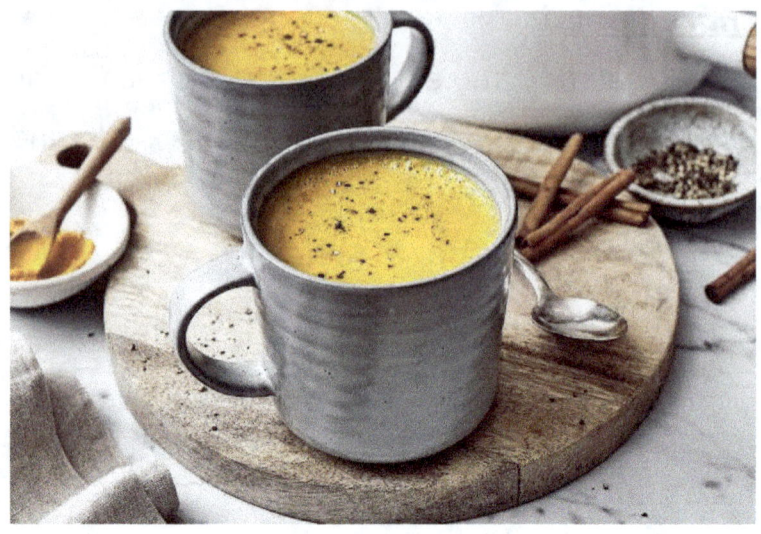

Ingredients:

- Turmeric powder
- Ground cinnamon
- Ground ginger
- Honey or maple syrup
- Coconut milk or almond milk

Procedure:

1. In a small saucepan, heat coconut milk or almond milk over medium heat.

2. Add turmeric powder, ground cinnamon, and ground ginger to the milk, stirring well.
3. Simmer the mixture for a few minutes to allow the flavors to meld together.
4. Sweeten with honey or maple syrup to taste.
5. Pour the golden milk into a mug and enjoy its warm and comforting properties.

These beverage recipes offer a variety of flavors and health benefits to complement your COPD management journey. Remember to adjust the ingredients and sweetness levels based on your preferences and dietary requirements. Staying hydrated with nourishing drinks not only supports your overall well-being but also helps maintain optimal lung health.

Chapter 8

Recipe Modifications

Adapting recipes to meet specific dietary needs and preferences is an important aspect of managing COPD. In this chapter, we will explore some recipe modifications and adaptations that can accommodate various dietary restrictions or personal choices while still providing delicious and nutritious meals.

Gluten-Free Options:

1. Substitute regular flour with gluten-free flours such as almond flour, coconut flour, or gluten-free all-purpose flour.
2. Use gluten-free breadcrumbs or crushed gluten-free cereal as a coating or topping.
3. Opt for gluten-free grains like quinoa, brown rice, or millet in place of wheat-based grains.

Dairy-Free Alternatives:

1. Replace cow's milk with plant-based milks such as almond milk, coconut milk, or oat milk.

2. Use dairy-free cheese substitutes made from soy, almond, or rice.

3. Replace butter with dairy-free spreads or oils like olive oil or coconut oil.

Low Sodium Modifications:

1. Reduce or omit salt from recipes and instead use herbs, spices, and citrus juices to enhance flavors.

2. Choose low-sodium or salt-free versions of ingredients like broths, canned beans, and condiments.

3. Opt for fresh or frozen vegetables instead of canned vegetables, which often contain added sodium.

Vegetarian or Vegan Adaptations:

1. Substitute meat with plant-based protein sources like tofu, tempeh, beans, lentils, or chickpeas.
2. Use vegetable broth instead of meat-based broths.
3. Incorporate plant-based oils or vegan butter substitutes in place of animal fats.

Allergen-Free Options:

1. Replace common allergens like nuts with seeds (e.g., sunflower seeds or pumpkin seeds) for added crunch or creaminess.
2. Use alternative sweeteners like maple syrup, agave nectar, or stevia for those with sugar allergies or restrictions.
3. Be mindful of individual allergens and make ingredient substitutions accordingly.

Portion Control:

1. Adjust portion sizes according to individual calorie and nutritional needs.
2. Use smaller plates and bowls to visually create the illusion of a fuller plate.
3. Include a variety of nutrient-dense foods to feel satisfied with smaller portions.

Remember to consult with a healthcare professional or registered dietitian for personalized dietary recommendations based on your specific needs. By making these recipe modifications, you can ensure that your meals align with your dietary preferences and requirements while supporting your COPD management journey.

Chapter 9

Cooking Techniques

Choosing the right cooking techniques can have a significant impact on the nutritional value and overall healthfulness of your meals, especially when managing COPD. In this chapter, we will explore some healthier cooking methods that can help retain nutrients, minimize the use of added fats, and enhance the flavors of COPD-friendly meals.

1. Steaming:

Steaming is a gentle cooking method that helps preserve the nutrients in foods while retaining their natural flavors and textures. It involves using steam to cook ingredients without submerging them in water. Steam vegetables, fish, or poultry by placing them in a steamer basket or steaming rack over simmering water.

Steaming is an excellent technique for preserving the lung-friendly nutrients in foods.

2. Grilling:

Grilling adds a smoky and charred flavor to foods without the need for excessive oils or fats. Use a gas or charcoal grill to cook lean meats, fish, vegetables, and even fruits. Marinate foods beforehand to enhance flavors and prevent dryness. Opt for lean cuts of meat and remove excess fat to promote a heart-healthy and COPD-friendly meal.

3. Stir-Frying:

Stir-frying involves quickly cooking small, bite-sized pieces of ingredients in a small amount of oil over high heat. This technique retains the natural colors, textures, and flavors of the ingredients while minimizing the cooking time. Use a non-stick pan or wok and a small amount of heart-healthy oil like olive oil or sesame oil.

Stir-fry vegetables, lean proteins, and whole grains to create flavorful and nutrient-rich meals.

4. Baking:

Baking is a dry-heat cooking method that is ideal for meats, poultry, fish, and even vegetables. It requires minimal added fats and helps retain the natural flavors and nutrients in the ingredients. Use parchment paper or non-stick baking pans to reduce the need for excessive oils. Add herbs, spices, and citrus juices to enhance the flavors of baked dishes without relying on unhealthy ingredients.

5. Roasting:

Roasting involves cooking ingredients in the oven at a high temperature. It brings out the natural sweetness and flavors of vegetables and meats. Use a minimal amount of heart-healthy oil, such as olive oil, to coat the ingredients and prevent sticking. Roast vegetables, chicken, turkey, or fish for a delicious and nutritious COPD-friendly meal.

6. Poaching:

Poaching is a gentle cooking method that involves simmering foods in a liquid such as water, broth, or even fruit juice. This technique helps retain the moisture and tenderness of the ingredients without adding excessive fats. Poach fish, poultry, or fruits for a healthy and flavorful meal option.

By utilizing these healthier cooking techniques, you can create flavorful and nutrient-rich meals while minimizing the use of unhealthy fats and oils. Experiment with different methods to discover your favorite cooking techniques that suit your COPD management goals and personal taste preferences.

Chapter 10

Practical Tips

Meal planning, grocery shopping, and food storage are essential aspects of managing COPD and ensuring a well-balanced diet. In this chapter, we will explore some practical tips to help you streamline your meal preparation process, make healthier food choices, and store ingredients properly to maintain their freshness.

Meal Planning:

1. Plan your meals for the week ahead to ensure a variety of balanced and nutritious options.
2. Consider your specific dietary needs and preferences when selecting recipes.

3. Include a mix of lean proteins, whole grains, fruits, and vegetables in your meal plan.
4. Prepare a shopping list based on your planned meals to avoid impulse purchases and ensure you have all the necessary ingredients on hand.

Grocery Shopping:

1. Stick to the perimeter of the grocery store, where fresh produce, lean proteins, and dairy products are typically located.
2. Read food labels to make informed choices about the nutritional content and avoid ingredients that may exacerbate COPD symptoms.
3. Choose fresh, seasonal produce whenever possible for optimal flavor and nutrient content.

4. Consider purchasing frozen fruits and vegetables as a convenient alternative that retains their nutritional value.

Food Storage:

1. Properly store perishable items like meat, poultry, and seafood in the refrigerator or freezer to prevent spoilage.
2. Use airtight containers or resealable bags to store leftovers and maintain their freshness.
3. Label and date items to ensure you use them before they expire.
4. Keep a well-organized pantry and refrigerator to easily identify ingredients and minimize waste.

Batch Cooking and Portioning:

1. Prepare larger quantities of meals and portion them into individual servings for easy grab-and-go options.

2. Use freezer-friendly containers or resealable bags to store pre-portioned meals in the freezer.
3. Thaw frozen meals in the refrigerator overnight or use a microwave or stovetop for quicker defrosting.

Cooking in Advance:

1. Dedicate specific times during the week to batch cook and prepare meals in advance.
2. Cook staple ingredients like grains, legumes, or proteins in larger quantities to use as a base for multiple meals.
3. Pre-cut vegetables and store them in the refrigerator for quicker meal preparation.

Stocking Essentials:

1. Keep a well-stocked pantry with staple items like whole grains, canned beans, broths, herbs, and spices.

2. Have a variety of healthy snacks on hand to avoid reaching for less nutritious options.
3. Consider investing in kitchen tools and appliances that make meal preparation more efficient, such as a slow cooker or food processor.
4. By incorporating these practical tips into your routine, you can streamline your meal planning, grocery shopping, and food storage processes, ensuring that you have the necessary ingredients and tools to support your COPD management and maintain a healthy diet.